Natural Antibiotics

Discover the Ancient Secrets to Treat
Disease and Cure Sickness

Table of Contents

Introduction

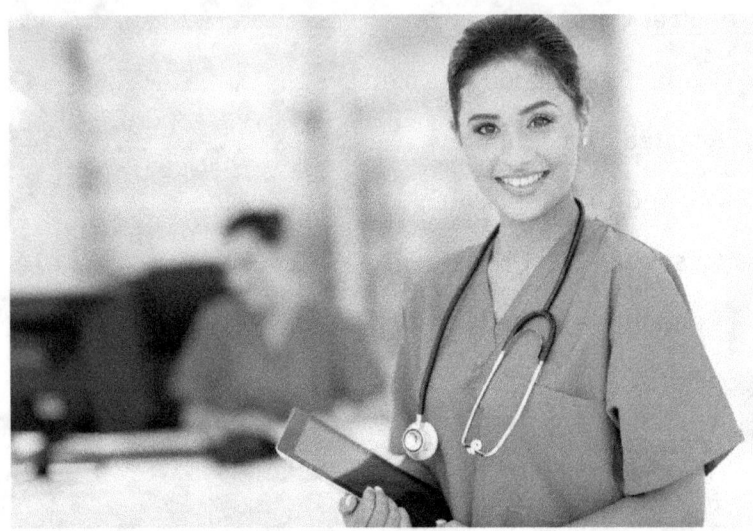

When you get sick, what do you usually do? If you are like most people, you probably make an appointment with your doctor or head to the local drug store for over-the-counter medications. Depending what you have come down with, you might be prescribed some kind of prescription medication. According to the CDC, nearly 50% of the United States population has used at least one prescription medication during the last thirty days and nearly 22% have used three or more prescriptions. Each year, regularly office physicians order a whopping 2.6 billion drugs and hospital emergency rooms order about 286 million more.

While it is true that medications can be very helpful in managing and curing certain conditions, they are not without their risks. Many medications come with nasty side effects that can sometimes be worse than the condition they are supposed to treat. Antibiotics are one of the most commonly prescribed medications, especially for things like cold and flu. Unfortunately, many people do not realize that certain strains of disease can actually become resistant to the effects of antibiotics – even if you take them as directed! Another problem with antibiotics is that while they work to destroy harmful bacteria, they can't tell the difference between good and bad so they can kill off the beneficial flora in your digestive tract as well. These effects are compounded when people do not finish the full course of their antibiotics, stopping early because they "feel better".

Although prescription antibiotics can be very bad for you and your body, not all antibiotics are bad. In fact, there are a number of foods that actually act as natural antibiotics. These natural antibiotics provide many of the same benefits as prescription antibiotics without destroying the good bacteria in your body. <u>Some examples of natural antibiotic foods and supplements are listed here below</u>:

- Grapefruit Seed Extract
- Echinacea
- Colloidal Silver
- Oregano Essential Oil

- Thyme Essential Oil
- Basil Essential Oil
- Lavender Essential Oil
- Garlic
- Onion
- Ginger
- Cayenne Pepper
- Curry Powder
- Turmeric
- Manuka Honey
- Cinnamon
- Cardamom

Now that you know the basics about natural antibiotics and have received a list of foods and supplements you may be eager to try them for yourself! If so, you will find a list of twenty-five recipes for natural antibiotics in the next section. Some of these recipes are for beverages, snacks, and meals that have natural antibiotic qualities and others are for natural remedies made using antibiotic essential oils.

Natural Antibiotic Recipes

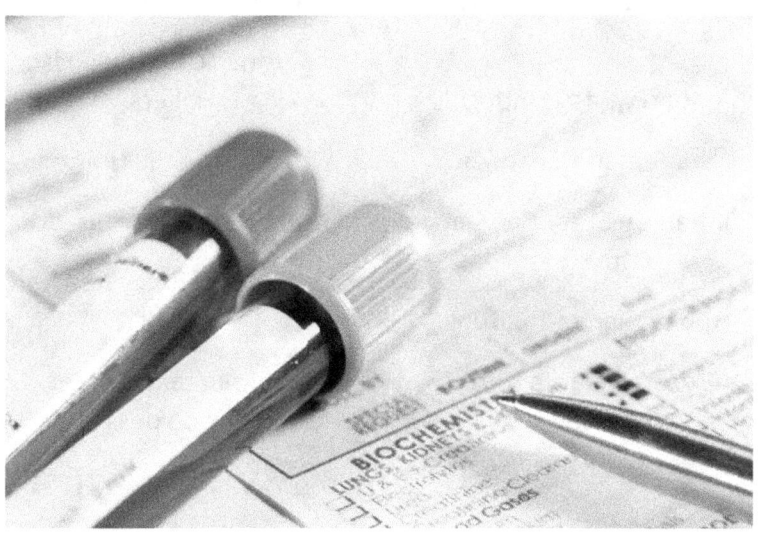

Recipes Included in this Book:

Echinacea Tincture for
Cold and Flu

Oregano Oil Soak for Foot
Fungus

Flu-Fighting Essential Oil
Blend

Oregano Inhalation for
Sinus Infections

Lemon, Ginger and
Manuka Honey Tea for
Cold/Flu

Massage Oil for Urinary
Tract Infections

Soothing Antibiotic Bath
Oil

Oil Blend for Strep Throat

Immune-Boosting Foot
Rub

Honey Cinnamon Blend
for Sore Throat

Daily Antibiotic Tonic

Carrot, Ginger and Beet Smoothie

Cinnamon Banana Oat Smoothie

Blueberry Basil Smoothie

Homemade Chai Tea

Cinnamon Steel-Cut Oats with Honey

Honey Cinnamon Buns

Roasted Garlic Herb Bread

Herb-Crusted Pork Tenderloin

Ginger Coconut Curry

Turmeric-Roasted Fish Fillets

Roasted Garlic Hummus

Almond-Ginger Biscotti

Sweet and Spicy Roasted Nuts

Homemade Ginger Cookies

Natural Antibiotic Oils and Supplements Recipes

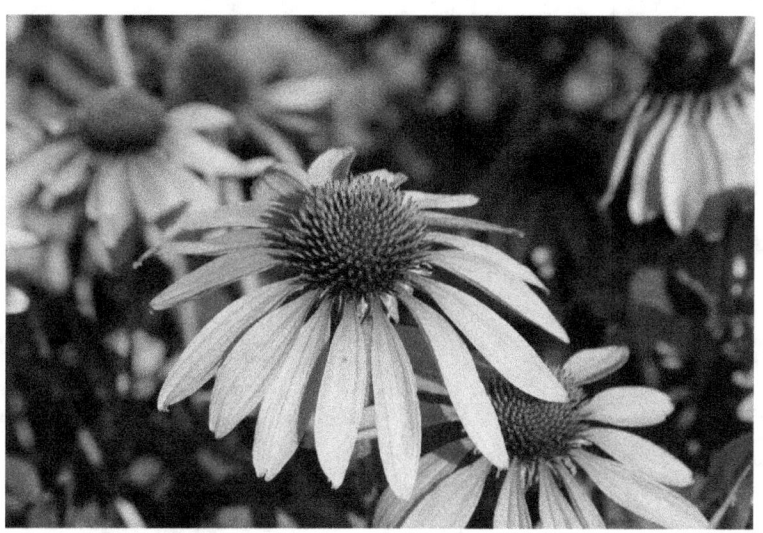

Echinacea Tincture for Cold and Flu

Ingredients:

- ¼ cup dried Echinacea
- 2 cups high-proof vodka

Instructions:

1. Place the dried Echinacea in a glass pint jar.
2. Pour in the vodka, filling the jar almost to the top.
3. Seal the jar with the lid and let it rest at room temperature for 4 to 6 weeks.

4. Strain the herbs out of the liquid and pour the liquid (the tincture) into a dark glass bottle.
5. Cover with the top and store in a cool, dark place.
6. Take 30 drops of the tincture by mouth once per hour until symptoms are gone.

Oregano Oil Soak for Foot Fungus

Ingredients:

- Hot water, as needed
- 2 teaspoons oregano essential oil
- Olive oil, optional

Instructions:

1. Fill a small tub with hot water and add the essential oil.
2. Swirl gently by hand to disperse the oil then soak your feet for 20 minutes.
3. Towel your feet dry and put on a warm pair of sock.
4. Alternatively, combine 1 teaspoon olive oil per 1 drop oregano essential oil.
5. Massage the oil blend into the nails or skin affected by the fungus.

Flu-Fighting Essential Oil Blend

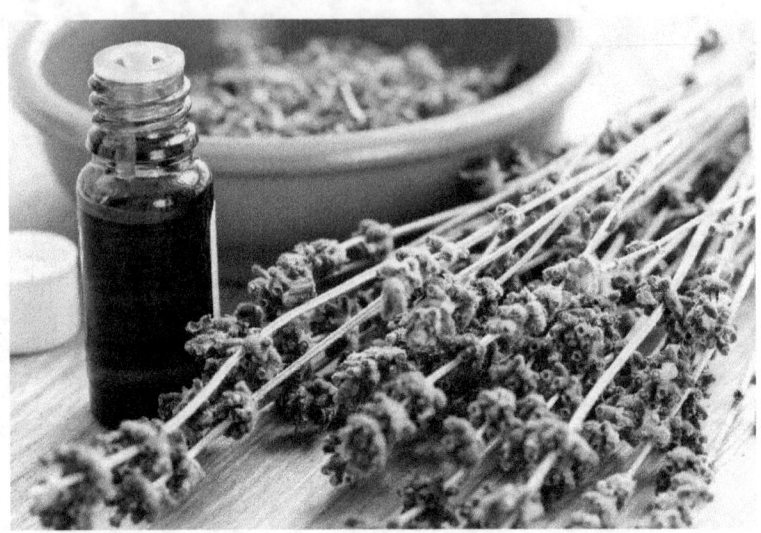

Ingredients:

- 24 drops thieves essential oil
- 12 drops lavender essential oil
- 4 drops frankincense essential oil

Instructions:

1. Combine the essential oils in a small dark glass bottle and swirl to combine.
2. Use an eye-dropper to fill empty gel capsules with the oil blend.
3. Take one capsule every 4 hours for three consecutive days.
4. Take on capsule every 8 hours for the next 4 to 6 days until the flu is gone.

Oregano Inhalation for Sinus Infections

Ingredients:

- Very hot water, as needed
- 3 to 5 drops oregano essential oil

Instructions:

1. Place a bowl of steaming water on the table.
2. Add the drops of oregano essential oil.
3. Lean over the bowl and cover your head and shoulders with a towel.
4. Breathe deeply to relieve sinus infection symptoms.

Lemon, Ginger and Manuka Honey Tea for Cold/Flu

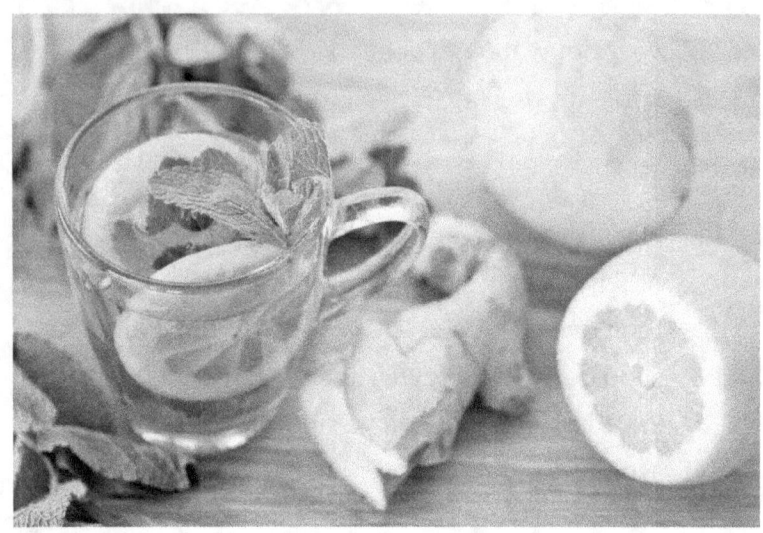

Ingredients:

- ½-inch piece ginger, peeled and sliced
- 1 teaspoon Manuka honey
- Hot water, as needed
- 1 to 2 drops ginger essential oil
- 1 to 2 tablespoons fresh lemon juice

Instructions:

1. Place the sliced ginger in a mug or teacup and mash it with a fork.
2. Add the honey then pour in the hot water and the essential oil.

3. Let the tea steep for 2 to 3 minutes then stir in the lemon juice.
4. Enjoy the tea while it is hot.

Massage Oil for Urinary Tract Infections

Ingredients:

- 1 teaspoon jojoba oil
- 3 to 4 drops mountain savory essential oil
- 2 drops lavender essential oil

Instructions:

1. Combine the oils in a small dark glass bottle and swirl to combine.
2. Massage a few drops of the oil blend into the skin on your abdomen, just above the pubic bone.
3. Repeat twice daily for three days until the infection is gone.

Soothing Antibiotic Bath Oil

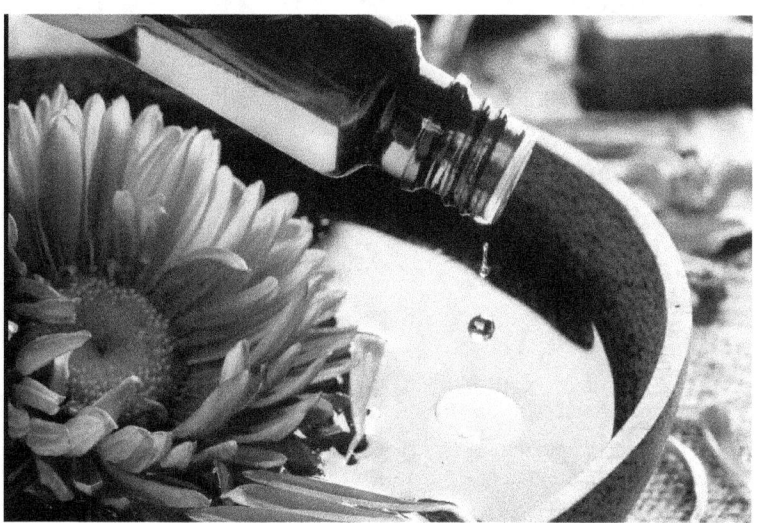

Ingredients:

- 1 cup sweet almond or jojoba oil
- 20 drops ginger essential oil
- 16 drops palmarosa essential oil
- 16 drops pine essential oil
- 14 drops lavender essential oil

Instructions:

1. Combine the oils in a small dark glass bottle and swirl to combine.
2. Put the stopper on the bottle and let it rest for 24 hours.
3. Run a hot bath then add 1 to 2 tablespoons of the oil blend to the water.

4. Swirl the water by hand to distribute the oils.
5. Soak for at least 20 minutes then towel dry and go to bed.

Oil Blend for Strep Throat

Ingredients:

- 18 drops thieves essential oil
- 10 to 12 drops oregano essential oil
- 4 drops frankincense essential oil

Instructions:

1. Combine the oils in a small dark glass bottle and swirl to combine.
2. Use an eye-dropper to fill empty gel capsules with the oil blend.
3. Take one capsule three times a day to relieve strep throat symptoms.
4. Additionally, rub a few drops of the blend into the bottoms of your feet once a day.

Immune-Boosting Foot Rub

Ingredients:

- 30 drops extra-virgin olive oil
- 15 drops oregano essential oil
- 15 drops eucalyptus essential oil
- 5 drops frankincense essential oil

Instructions:

1. Combine the oils in a small dark glass bottle and swirl to combine.
2. Rub several drops of the mixture into the soles of your feet to boost immunity.

Honey Cinnamon Blend for Sore Throat

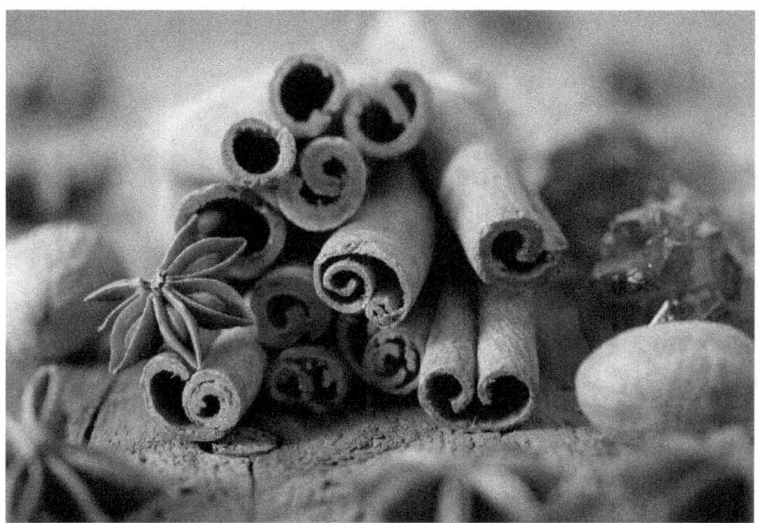

Ingredients:

- 1 cup Manuka honey
- ½ to 1 teaspoon ground cinnamon

Instructions:

1. Pour the honey into a small glass jar.
2. Stir in the cinnamon then cover the jar and let rest for 24 hours.
3. Take the mixture by mouth one tablespoon at a time to soothe sore throat and cough.
4. As an alternative, blend with hot water to create a soothing tea.

Natural Antibiotics Food Recipes

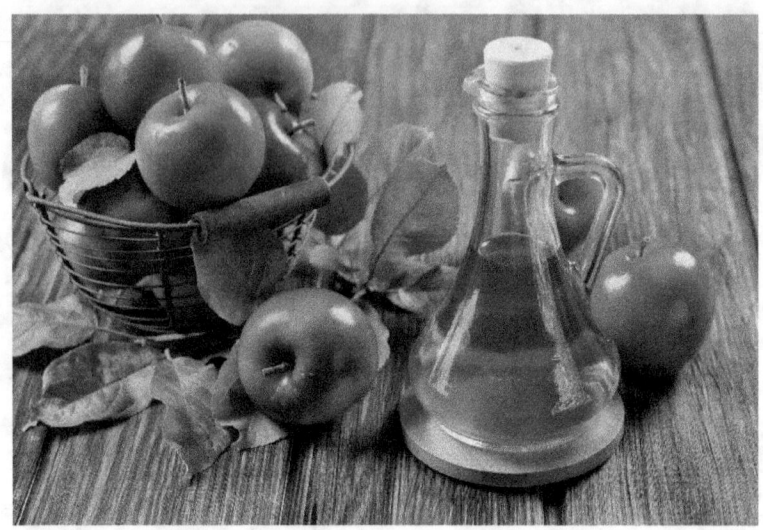

Daily Antibiotic Tonic

Servings: Makes about 3 cups

Ingredients:

- 2 cups organic apple cider vinegar
- 2 tablespoons fresh minced garlic
- 2 tablespoons fresh grated ginger
- 2 tablespoons diced onion
- ½ habanero pepper, seeded and minced
- 1 tablespoon fresh grated horseradish
- 1 tablespoon fresh chopped turmeric

Instructions:

1. Combine all of the ingredients in a high-speed blender.
2. Blend on high speed for 2 to 3 minutes then strain the liquid.
3. Store the liquid in a glass jar or bottle with the lid on.
4. Take 1 tablespoon by mouth daily for immunity – increase dosage for cold/flu.

Carrot, Ginger and Beet Smoothie

Servings: 1 to 2

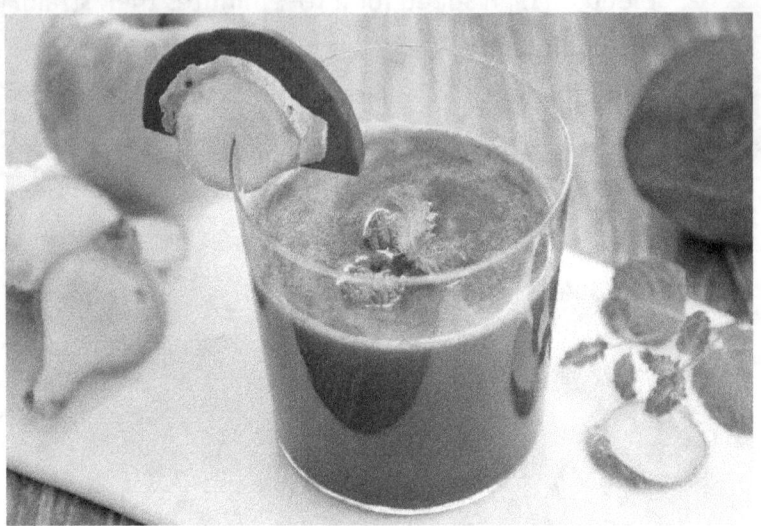

Ingredients:

- 1 small beet, peeled and chopped
- 1 small apple, cored, peeled and chopped
- 1 small carrot, peeled and chopped
- 1 ½ cups cold water (more, if needed)
- 1 to 2 tablespoons fresh lemon juice
- 1 handful fresh chopped kale
- 1 teaspoon fresh grated ginger
- 1 teaspoon Manuka honey

Instructions:

1. Combine all of the ingredients in a high-speed blender.

2. Pulse the ingredients several times to combine.
3. Blend on high speed for 30 to 60 seconds until blended.
4. Pour the smoothie into a glass and enjoy immediately.

Cinnamon Banana Oat Smoothie

Servings: 1

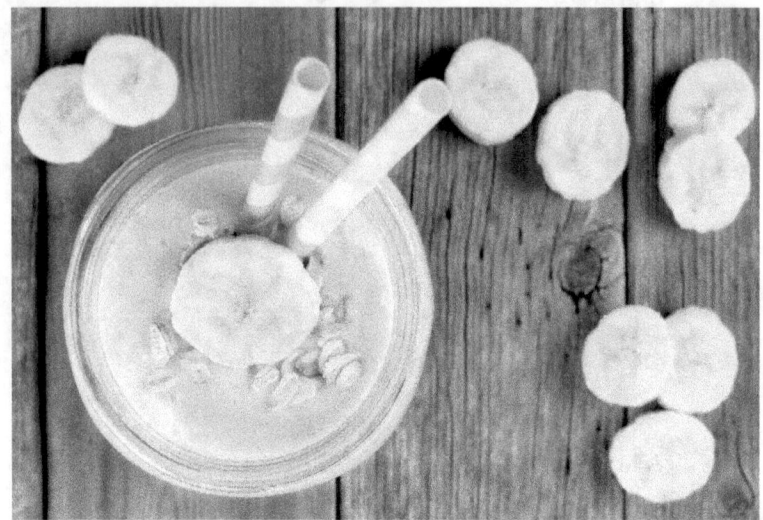

Ingredients:

- 1 medium frozen banana, peeled and chopped
- ¾ cup nonfat Greek yogurt, plain
- ½ cup fat-free milk
- ¼ cup old-fashioned oats
- ½ tablespoon Manuka honey
- ¼ teaspoon ground cinnamon

Instructions:

1. Combine all of the ingredients in a high-speed blender.
2. Pulse the ingredients several times to combine.
3. Blend on high speed for 30 to 60 seconds until blended.

4. Pour the smoothie into a glass and enjoy
    immediately.

Blueberry Basil Smoothie

Servings: 1

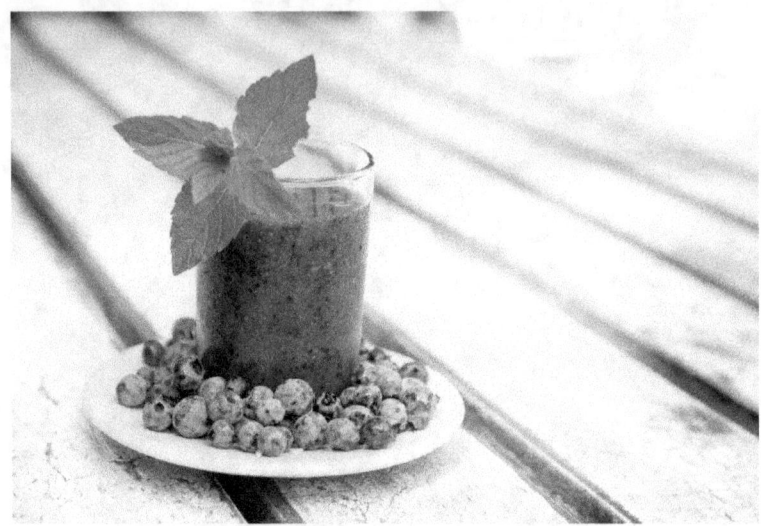

Ingredients:

- 1 ½ cups frozen blueberries
- ½ small frozen banana, peeled and chopped
- 1 ½ cups fat-free milk
- ½ cup nonfat Greek yogurt, plain
- ¼ cup fresh chopped basil
- 1 teaspoon Manuka honey
- Pinch ground ginger

Instructions:

1. Combine all of the ingredients in a high-speed blender.
2. Pulse the ingredients several times to combine.

3. Blend on high speed for 30 to 60 seconds until blended.
4. Pour the smoothie into a glass and enjoy immediately.

Homemade Chai Tea

Servings: 4 to 6

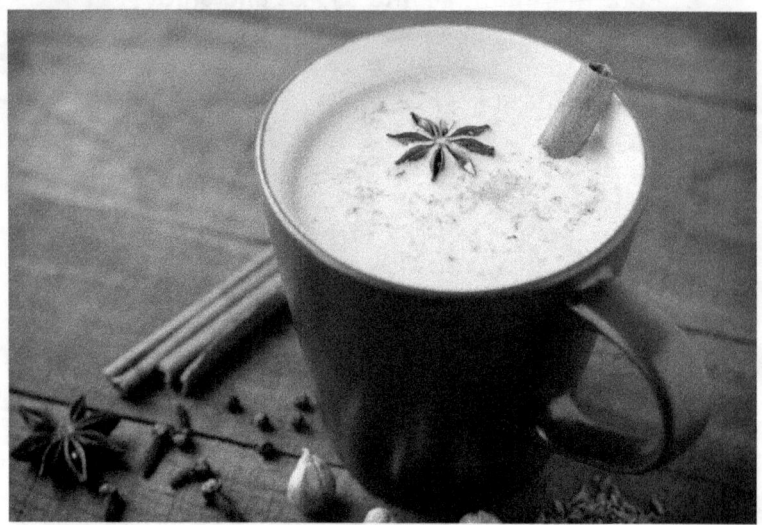

Ingredients:

- 2 tablespoons fresh grated ginger
- 2 cinnamon sticks, broken into pieces
- ½ tablespoon black peppercorns
- 10 cloves, whole
- 6 cardamom pods
- 6 cups filtered water
- 6 black tea bags
- 2 cups whole milk
- ¼ to ½ cup brown sugar, packed

Instructions:

1. Combine all of the spices in a medium saucepan.

2. Crush the spices gently with a wooden spoon then pour in the water.

3. Bring the mixture to a boil then reduce heat and simmer, partially covered, for 10 to 12 minutes.

4. Remove the saucepan from the heat and add the tea bags.

5. Steep the tea for 4 to 5 minutes then discard them.

6. Add the milk and sugar then simmer until the sugar is dissolved.

7. Strain the mixture and serve hot.

Cinnamon Steel-Cut Oats with Honey

Servings: 4 to 6

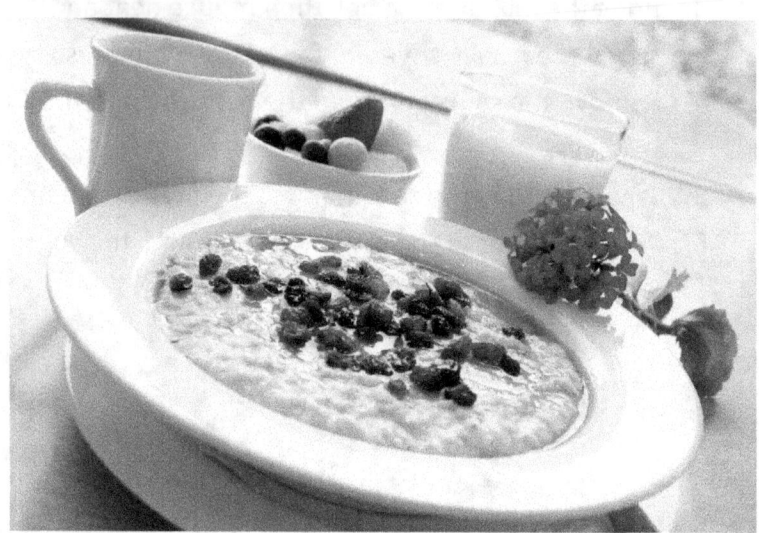

Ingredients:

- 1 tablespoon unsalted butter
- 1 ½ cups steel-cut oats
- 5 cups boiling water
- 1 to 1 ½ cups whole milk or buttermilk
- 2 tablespoons Manuka honey
- ½ teaspoon ground cinnamon

Instructions:

1. Melt the butter in a large saucepan over medium heat then stir in the oats.
2. Cook the oats for about 2 minutes until toasted.
3. Pour in the boiling water then simmer the oats for 25 minutes until tender.

4. Stir in the milk, honey and cinnamon then spoon into bowls to serve.

Honey Cinnamon Buns

Servings: 12

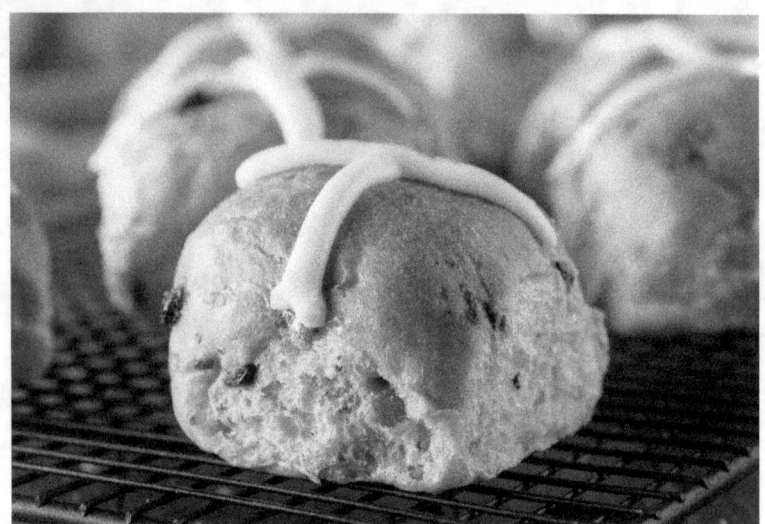

Ingredients:

- 1 lbs. frozen bread dough, thawed
- ¼ cup Manuka honey
- ¼ cup chopped nuts, toasted
- 2 tablespoons salted butter, softened
- 1 teaspoon ground cinnamon

Instructions:

1. Preheat the oven to 375°F and grease a muffin pan with cooking spray.
2. Roll the bread dough out on a lightly floured surface into a large rectangle.
3. In a bowl, stir together the honey, chopped nuts, butter and cinnamon.

4. Spread the mixture over the dough then roll it up into a log.

5. Cut the log into 12 slices and place one in each cup of the prepared muffin pan.

6. Let the dough rise for 30 minutes then bake for 20 minutes until golden brown.

Roasted Garlic Herb Bread

Servings: makes 1 loaf

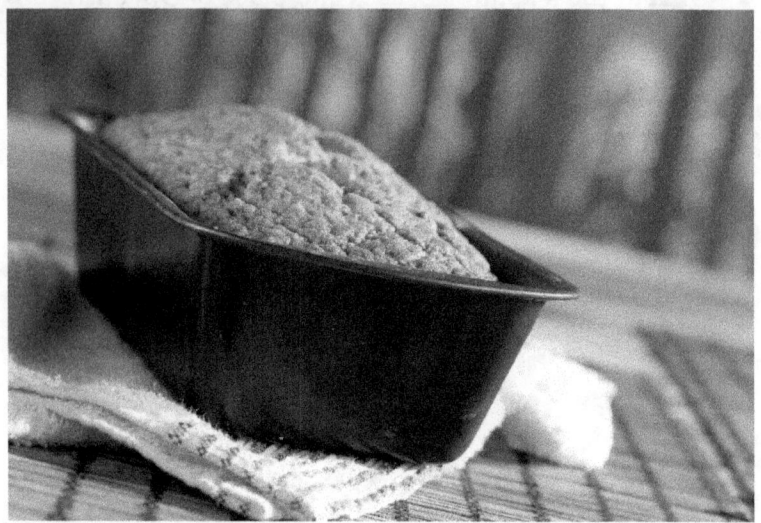

Ingredients:

- 1 ½ cups white whole-wheat flour
- 1 cup all-purpose flour
- 2 tablespoons dried herbs (your choice)
- 3 teaspoons baking powder
- ½ teaspoon baking soda
- ½ teaspoon salt
- 1 ¼ cups fat-free milk
- 6 tablespoons olive oil
- 2 large eggs, beaten well

Instructions:

1. Preheat the oven to 375°F and grease a loaf pan with cooking spray.
2. Combine the flours, herbs, baking soda, baking powder, and salt in a mixing bowl.
3. In a separate bowl, whisk together the milk, eggs, and olive oil.
4. Stir the wet ingredients into the dry until just combined.
5. Fold in the garlic then spoon the batter into the prepared pan.
6. Bake for 40 to 45 minutes until a knife inserted in the center comes out clean.
7. Cool the bread for 15 minutes then turn out onto a wire rack to cool completely.

Herb-Crusted Pork Tenderloin

Servings: 6 to 8

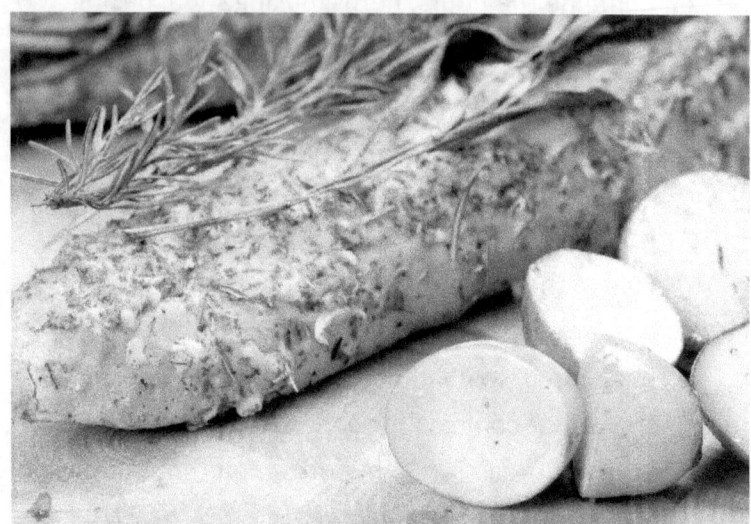

Ingredients:

- 1 (4 to 4 ½ lbs.) boneless pork tenderloin
- Salt and pepper to taste
- 2 tablespoons olive oil
- 1 tablespoon minced garlic
- 2 teaspoons fresh chopped thyme
- 2 teaspoons fresh chopped rosemary
- 2 teaspoons fresh chopped basil
- 1 teaspoon fresh chopped oregano

Instructions:

1. Preheat the oven to 475°F.

2. Place the pork fat-side-up in a roasting pan and season with salt and pepper to taste.

3. Stir together the olive oil, garlic, and herbs in a small bowl.

4. Rub the mixture into the pork tenderloin on all sides.

5. Roast for about 30 minutes then reduce the oven temperature to 425°F.

6. Let the tenderloin roast for another 50 to 60 minutes until the internal temperature reaches 155°F.

7. Remove the pork to a cutting board and tent loosely with foil.

8. Let rest for 20 minutes then slice to serve.

Ginger Coconut Curry

Servings: 6 to 8

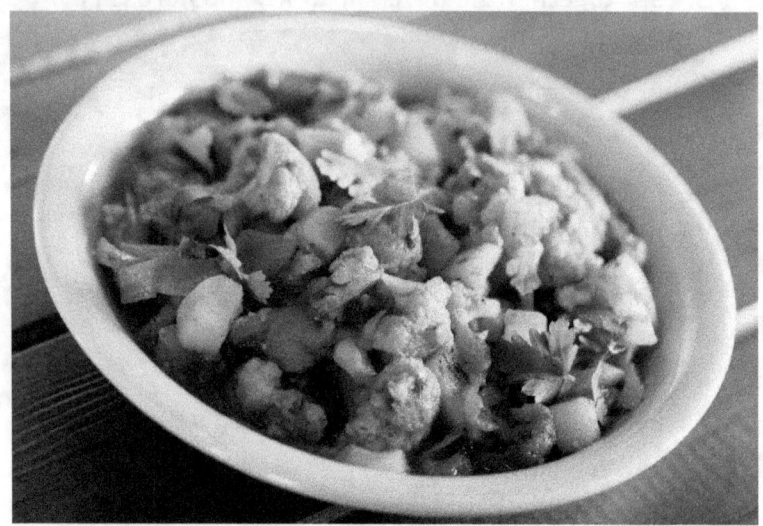

Ingredients:

- 1 tablespoon olive oil
- 1 medium yellow onion, chopped
- 1 teaspoon fresh grated ginger
- 1 teaspoon minced garlic
- 2 (14-ounce) cans coconut milk
- 2 tablespoons curry powder
- 1 teaspoon ground turmeric
- 2 tablespoons Manuka honey
- Salt to taste
- 2 large sweet potatoes, peeled and chopped
- 2 cups fresh chopped cauliflower florets
- 1 medium red pepper, cored and diced

- Fresh chopped cilantro, to serve

Instructions:

1. Heat the oil in a large saucepan over medium heat.
2. Add the onions, ginger and garlic and cook for 5 minutes, stirring often, until tender.
3. Stir in the coconut milk, curry powder, turmeric, honey and salt.
4. Bring the mixture to a simmer then stir in the sweet potatoes.
5. Simmer the sweet potatoes, covered, for 5 minutes then stir in the remaining vegetables.
6. Cover and steam for 5 to 10 minutes until the vegetables are tender.
7. Serve hot garnished with fresh cilantro.

Turmeric-Roasted Fish Fillets

Servings: 4

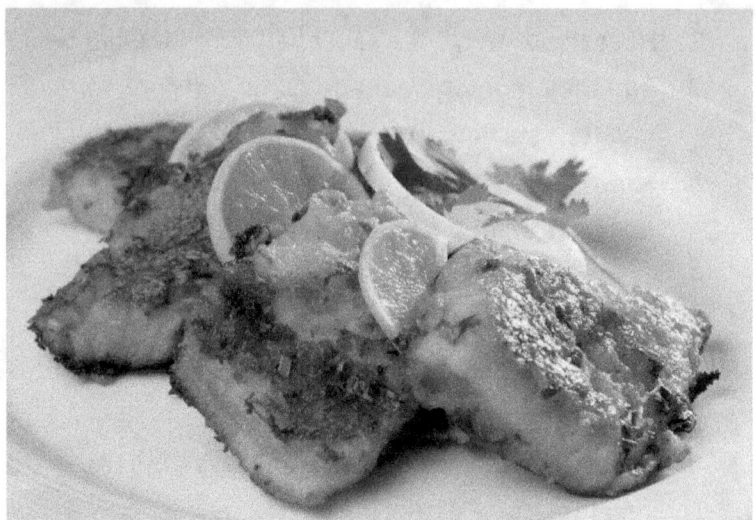

Ingredients:

- 3 teaspoons olive oil, divided
- 1 medium yellow onion, diced
- 1 teaspoon fresh grated ginger
- 1 teaspoon fresh minced garlic
- 1 cup long-grain white rice, uncooked
- 1 ½ cups low-sodium vegetable broth
- 1 tablespoon lemon juice
- 1 (15-ounce) can brown lentils, drained and rinsed
- 1 ½ teaspoons ground turmeric
- 1 teaspoon chili powder
- ½ teaspoon ground cumin
- ¼ teaspoon cayenne

- Salt and pepper to taste
- 4 (4 to 6-ounce) whitefish fillets, skin removed

Instructions:

1. Heat 1 teaspoon olive oil in a large saucepan over medium heat.
2. Stir in the onion, ginger and garlic then cook for 5 minutes until softened.
3. Add the rice then stir in the vegetable broth and lemon juice.
4. Bring the mixture to a boil then reduce heat and simmer for 10 minutes, covered, until the rice is tender.
5. Stir in the lentils and cook until heated through – about 5 minutes - then set side.
6. Combine the remaining oil with the turmeric, chili powder, cumin and cayenne in a small bowl.
7. Season the fillets with salt and pepper to taste then coat in the spice mixture.
8. Heat a large nonstick skillet over high heat and add the fillets.
9. Cook for 1 to 2 minutes on each side until just cooked through then serve with rice.

Roasted Garlic Hummus

Servings: makes about 1 ½ cups

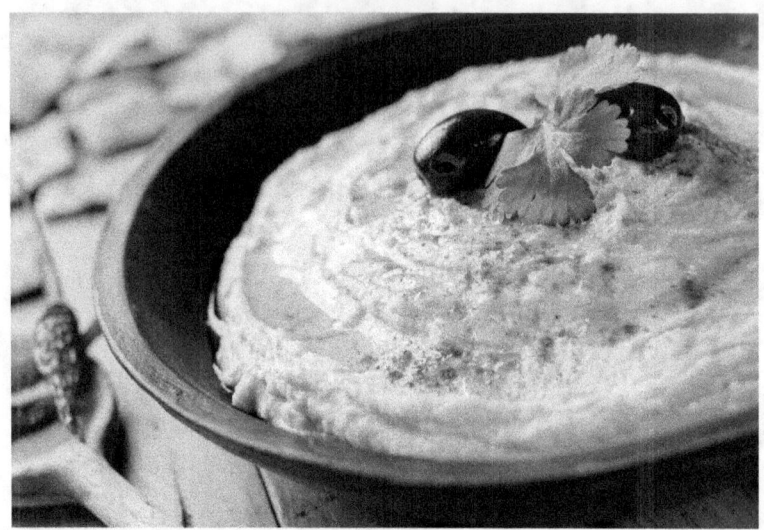

Ingredients:

- 1 head garlic, papery peel removed
- 1 (15-ounce) can chickpeas, rinsed and drained
- ¼ cup sesame tahini sauce
- 3 to 4 tablespoons fresh lemon juice
- Salt and pepper to taste
- 2 to 4 tablespoons olive oil
- Paprika, to serve
- Cayenne, to serve

Instructions:

1. Preheat the oven to 350°F.

2. Cut the top off a head of peeled garlic and place it on a piece of foil.
3. Drizzle with olive oil then wrap into a foil packet.
4. Roast the garlic for 45minutes until soft then let cool 10 minutes.
5. Squeeze the garlic cloves out of the head and set aside half of them.
6. Combine the chickpeas, tahini, and lemon juice in a food processor.
7. Add the salt, pepper and reserved garlic cloves.
8. Blend until smooth and well combined.
9. While blending, drizzle in the oil until the desired consistency is reached.
10. Spoon into a bowl and sprinkle with paprika and cayenne to serve.

Almond-Ginger Biscotti

Servings: 18 to 24

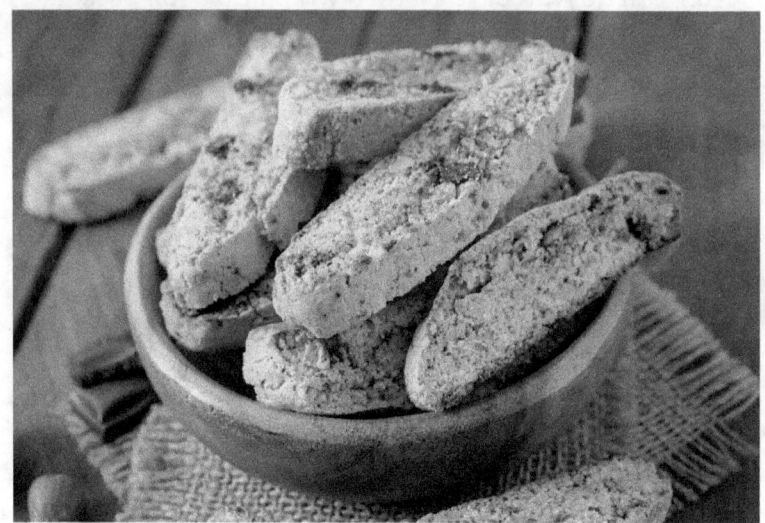

Ingredients:

- ¾ cups white granulated sugar
- ½ cup unsalted butter, softened
- ½ cup molasses
- 3 large eggs, beaten well
- ¼ cup fresh grated ginger
- 3 cups all-purpose flour
- 1 ¼ teaspoon ground cinnamon
- 1 teaspoon baking powder
- ½ teaspoon ground cloves
- ½ teaspoon ground allspice
- 1 cup toasted almonds

Instructions:

1. Preheat the oven to 350°F and line a baking sheet with parchment and dust with flour.
2. Beat together the sugar, butter and molasses in a bowl until creamy.
3. Add the eggs one at a time, beating between each addition, then stir in the ginger.
4. In a separate bowl, whisk together the flour, cinnamon, baking powder, cloves and allspice.
5. Add the dry ingredients to the wet until well combined then fold in the almonds.
6. Turn out the dough onto a floured surface and divide it in half.
7. Shape each half into a 10-inch log about 2 inches wide.
8. Place the logs on the baking sheet and bake for 30 minutes.
9. Cool the logs slightly then slice them diagonally and place the slices back on the baking sheet.
10. Bake for another 15 to 18 minutes until browned then cool completely.

Sweet and Spicy Roasted Nuts

Servings: makes 2 ½ cups

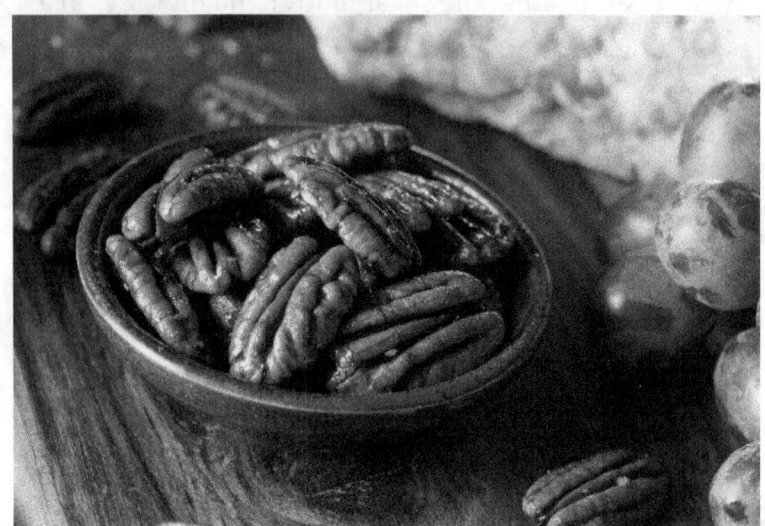

Ingredients:

- 2 cups whole almonds
- 1 ½ cups raw walnut haves
- 1 ½ cups pecan halves
- ½ cup raw cashews, whole
- ½ cup Manuka honey
- 3 tablespoons olive oil
- 2 teaspoons ground cinnamon
- ¼ teaspoon cayenne pepper
- 1 teaspoon salt

Instructions:

1. Preheat the oven to 300°F and line a baking sheet with foil.
2. Combine the nuts in a bowl with the honey, oil and spices.
3. Toss to coat then spread on the baking sheet and sprinkle with salt.
4. Bake for 45 minutes, stirring occasionally, until the nuts are golden brown.
5. Cool the nuts completely then store in an airtight container.

Homemade Ginger Cookies

Servings: 2 dozen

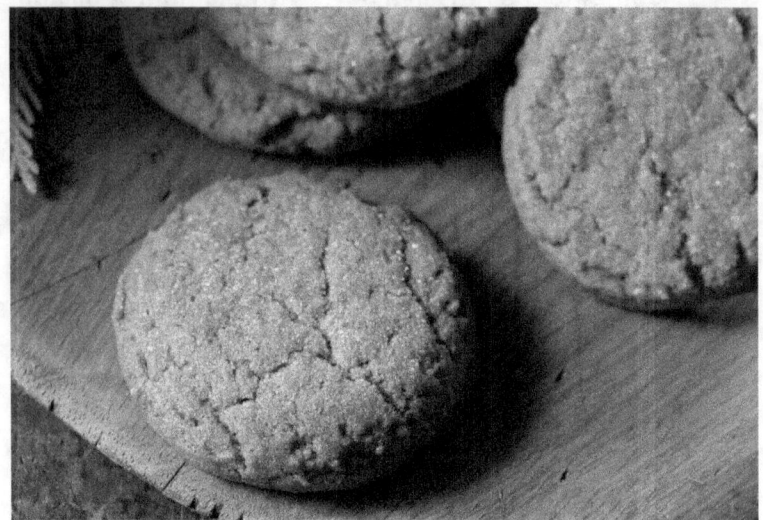

Ingredients:

- 4 ½ cups all-purpose flour
- ½ tablespoon baking soda
- 1 tablespoon ground ginger
- 1 ½ teaspoon ground cinnamon
- ¾ teaspoon ground cloves
- ½ teaspoon salt
- 3 sticks unsalted butter, softened
- 2 ¾ cups white sugar, divided
- 2 large eggs, beaten well
- ½ cup dark molasses

Instructions:

1. Preheat the oven to 350°F and line a baking sheet with parchment.
2. Combine the flour, baking soda, and spices in a mixing bowl.
3. In a separate bowl, beat together the butter with 2 cups of sugar until light and fluffy.
4. Beat in the eggs and molasses then stir in the dry ingredients.
5. Pinch off pieces of dough and roll them into 2-inch balls by hand.
6. Place the remaining sugar in a boll and roll the dough balls in it.
7. Place the balls on the baking sheet 2 inches apart then bake for 12 to 14 minutes until browned.

Conclusion

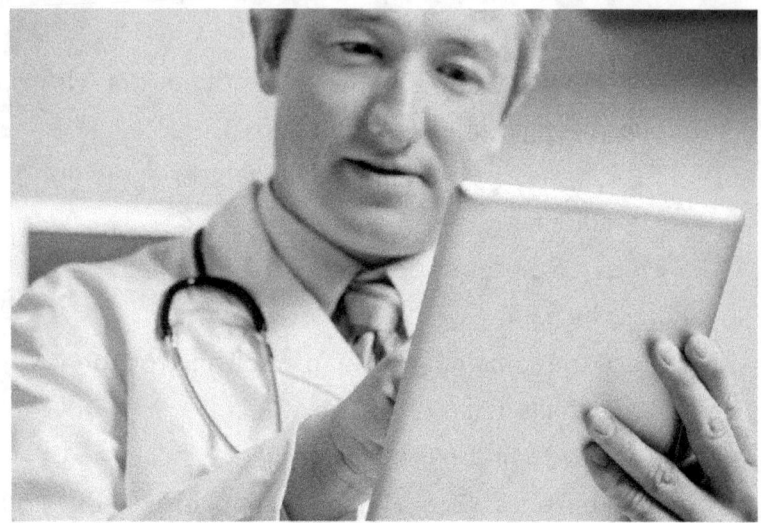

Popping a few pills to get rid of an infection may seem simple enough, but what is actually happening in your body could be completely different. Prescription antibiotics may work to kill off bad bacteria, but they can also destroy the good bacteria in your gut that are responsible for regulating your digestion. If you want to receive the benefits of antibiotics without the side effects, consider using natural antibiotic foods and supplements instead. To get you started, try out some of the wonderful recipes provided in this book! You will be amazed at the results and how simple they are to use.

www.ingramcontent.com/pod-product-compliance
Lightning Source LLC
Chambersburg PA
CBHW071254280526
45788CB00004B/1713